My 12 Week Training Log

KEEP TRACK, MAKE PROGRESS

I0450012

Wilberto Burgos Jr

Thank You for making the choice to use this journal on your new 12 week journey.

This 12 Week Training Log was designed with you in mind. Enter all of your information in one easy to carry book.

- Goals -
- Training Schedule -
- Appointments-
- Notes -
- Contact List -
- Supplement log -
- Measurement tracking -
- Food Log -
- Resistance training -
- Cardio training -

Wether you are an athlete, fitness buff or someone trying to better themselves in the quality of their lives, This 12 Week Training Log will help you keep track of all or your daily tasks and your progress.

Thanks Again for choosing My 12 Week Training Log

If you need any assistance or have any questions on how to use this log, send me an email: wilberto.burgos@yahoo.com

Setting Goals

Goal Setting is serious business, or at least it should be. Don't get all worked up and nervous. Just pay close attention to what you really want to accomplish and your goals will be reached. Follow these 8 simple rules and you will find that your goals are easier to meet than you thought.

Your Goals should be short and realistic (example, loose 5 pounds of fat by the end of my first two weeks.) Set your first Goal for two weeks, then four weeks, then 6 weeks = twelve weeks.

Set two long term Goals, each for six weeks = twelve weeks.
Good Luck on reaching your goals

•Create a plan•	•Write it down•
•Track progress•	•Be committed to yourself•
•Plan meals•	•Reward yourself•
•Avoid Gimmicks and Gadgets•	•If you need help, ask for it•

Notes

MY GOALS

Activity	Current	Goal	Start	End

Staying On Target

Yea, sometimes staying on target can be somewhat difficult,
But if you keep your mind set on your goals, you WILL accomplish them.

Make sure to set Realistic Short term goals, Plan out your next few weeks of exercise and it will all go smoothly.

Work on your schedule before you go to the gym and then change it when your their. Before you know-it, you will have your training schedule and your exercise program down to a science.

Listen to your body, when your sick, stay home, when you feel like just sitting at home in front of the T.V, get up and go for a walk.

Plan out the day to come before you goto bed and it will come close to what you set it to be.

Good Luck and keep your goals in the front of your mind.

Remember,
resistance training helps enhance bone density, helping to prevent osteoporosis.

Can't manage to complete a goal?
•Don't get discouraged•
•Recognize a partial accomplishment•
•Reassess your goals and change them•

Many people give up too soon
•Don't ever give up trying•
•If you fall behind, refocus•

Notes

he act of giving or getting nourishment)

o obtain food and use it for growth, metabolism, and repair.
he 6 stages of nutrition include ingestion, digestion, absorption,
:ansport, assimilation, and excretion.

•1 Kilogram is equal to 1,000 grams or 2.2 pounds•

Athletes should consume
between 6 and 7 grams of carbs per kilo of total body weight per day.

Calculating Protein needs
•1.4 grams per lean body weight for endurance•
•1.7 grams per lean body weight for muscle building•

Converting pounds to kilograms
•body weight divided by 2.2 = kg•
(ex...110 lbs divided by 2.2 = 50kg)

Remember, the body can not burn fat without carbs.

Try to include protein, carbs and fat in all of your meals.

•Nutrition should be the most important part of your training program•
•Nutrient timing is the key to successful goal completion•

)rink lots of water (64 ounces per day) since this is the most neglected, taken
iutrient the body needs to perform at greater levels.

Try to avoid the Magic diet pill or the Miracle muscle builder.
Most fad diets don't last the distance of your desired goal.
Keep a close eye on the Protein, Carbohydrate and Fat intake of your diet
as this will make all the difference on your fat loss and muscle gain. Food
timing is just one key to making it to your goal. Moderation is another key
to a healthier diet. To loose weight, burn more calories than you consume,
to gain more weight, burn less.

Good Luck on reaching your goals

Training Schedule

MONDAY

MUSCLE	EXERCISE	SETS	REPS

TUESDAY

MUSCLE	EXERCISE	SETS	REPS

Training Schedule

WEDNESDAY

MUSCLE	EXERCISE	SETS	REPS

THURSDAY

MUSCLE	EXERCISE	SETS	REPS

Training Schedule

FRIDAY

MUSCLE	EXERCISE	SETS	REPS

SATURDAY

MUSCLE	EXERCISE	SETS	REPS

Training Schedule

MUSCLE	EXERCISE	SETS	REPS

NOTES

Training Schedule / Appointments

Date	Schedule / Appointments	Time	Notes

Training Schedule / Appointments

Date	Schedule / Appointments	Time	Notes

NOTES

NOTES

NOTES

Contact List

Name: _____

Address: _____

City: _____ State: _____ Zip: _____

Phone: _____ E-Mail: _____

Name: _____

Address: _____

City: _____ State: _____ Zip: _____

Phone: _____ E-Mail: _____

Name: _____

Address: _____

City: _____ State: _____ Zip: _____

Phone: _____ E-Mail: _____

Name: _____

Address: _____

City: _____ State: _____ Zip: _____

Phone: _____ E-Mail: _____

Name: _____

Address: _____

City: _____ State: _____ Zip: _____

Phone: _____ E-Mail: _____

Name: _____

Address: _____

City: _____ State: _____ Zip: _____

Phone: _____ E-Mail: _____

Name: _____

Address: _____

City: _____ State: _____ Zip: _____

Phone: _____ E-Mail: _____

Name: _____

Address: _____

City: _____ State: _____ Zip: _____

Phone: _____ E-Mail: _____

Contact List

Name: _____

Address: _____

City: _____ State: _____ Zip: _____

Phone: _____ E-Mail: _____

Name: _____

Address: _____

City: _____ State: _____ Zip: _____

Phone: _____ E-Mail: _____

Name: _____

Address: _____

City: _____ State: _____ Zip: _____

Phone: _____ E-Mail: _____

Name: _____

Address: _____

City: _____ State: _____ Zip: _____

Phone: _____ E-Mail: _____

Name: _____

Address: _____

City: _____ State: _____ Zip: _____

Phone: _____ E-Mail: _____

Name: _____

Address: _____

City: _____ State: _____ Zip: _____

Phone: _____ E-Mail: _____

Name: _____

Address: _____

City: _____ State: _____ Zip: _____

Phone: _____ E-Mail: _____

Name: _____

Address: _____

City: _____ State: _____ Zip: _____

Phone: _____ E-Mail: _____

Supplements

Kind	Serving Size	Times per Day	Date

Supplements

Kind	Serving Size	Times per Day	Date

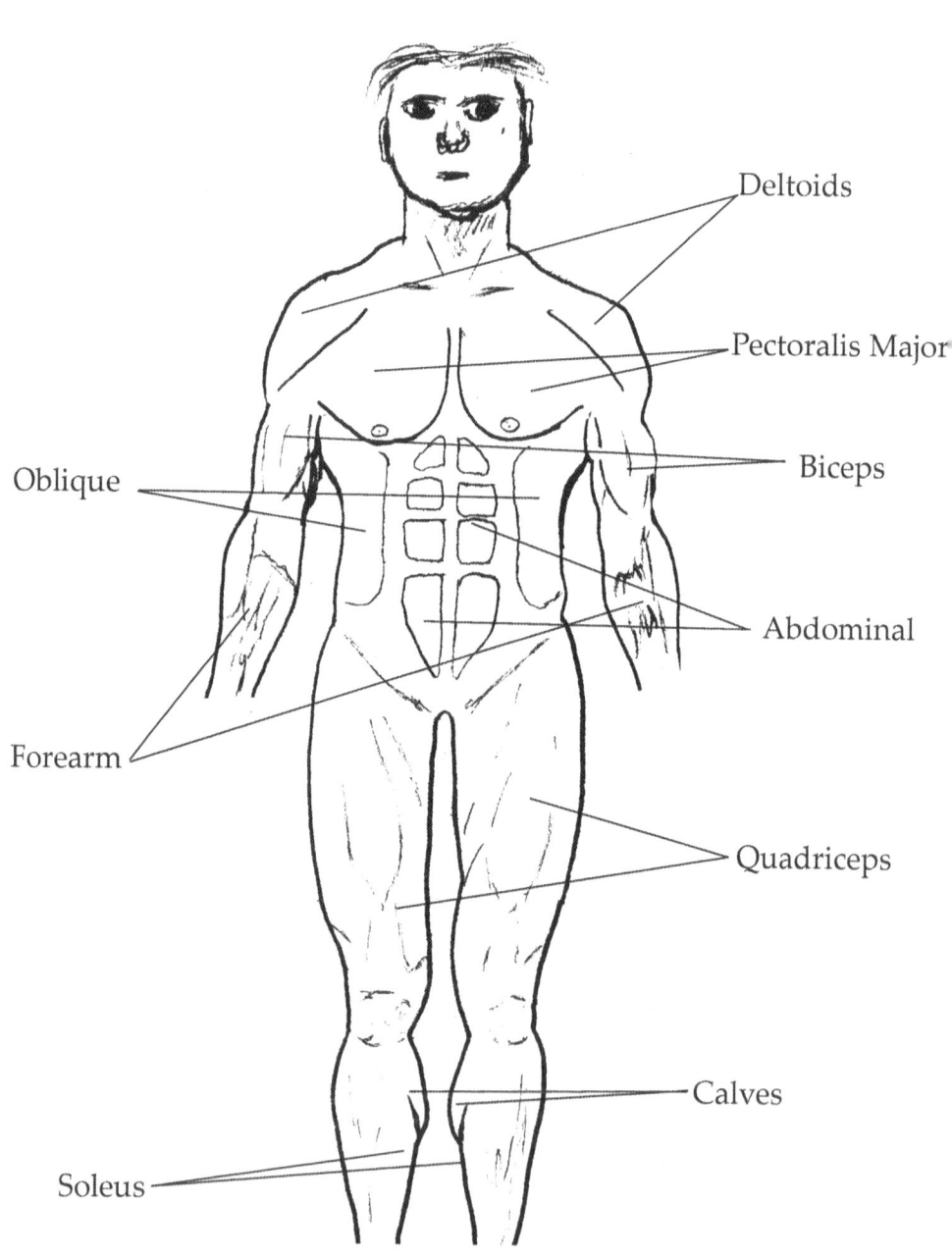

Deltoids

Pectoralis Major

Biceps

Oblique

Abdominal

Forearm

Quadriceps

Calves

Soleus

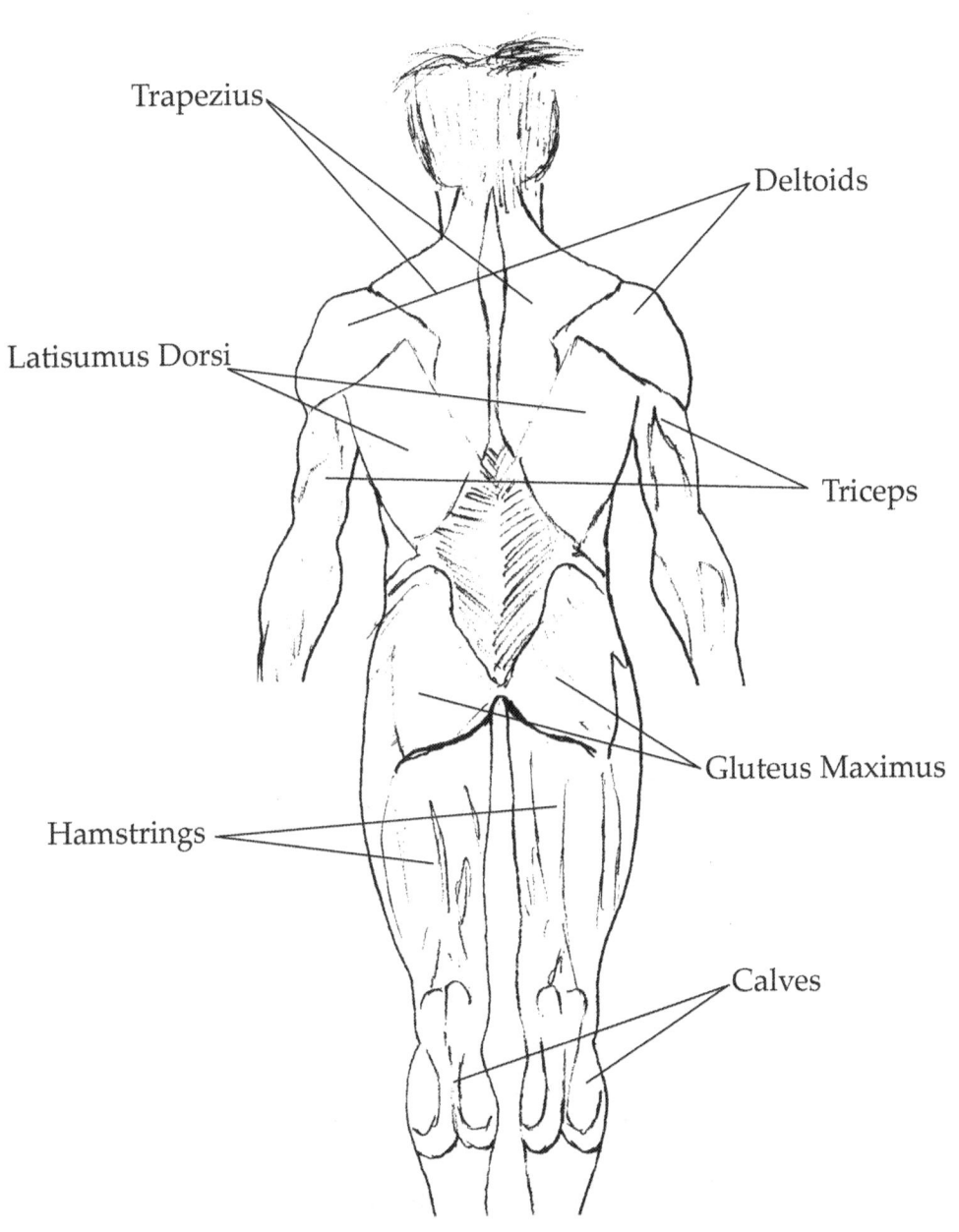

Trapezius

Deltoids

Latisumus Dorsi

Triceps

Gluteus Maximus

Hamstrings

Calves

Measurements

Date: _____/_____/_____ .... Start Date

Resting Heart Rate: - beats per minute -	
Target Heart Rate: - beats per minute -	LO _____ | HI _____

Neck	Chest	UpperArm	Waist	Hips
in.	in.	in.	in.	in.

Thigh	Calf	Forearm	Weight	Body Fat
in.	in.	in.	in.	%

The best time to find out your resting heart rate is in the morning, before you get out of bed.

The heart beats about 60 to 80 times a minute when we're at rest.

To calculate your resting heart rate, before you get out of bed check for your pulse then once you find it count it for 10 seconds then times that number by 6. This is your true resting heart rate.

To find your target heart rate minus your age from 220.
The number you get here must be set up for your high and lo heart rate.
The way you do this is by taking the number you just got and for the lo times it by .55, and for the high, times it by .85.

If you are are an endurance athlete times it by .95
and this will be your high.
Your lo can be times by .65.

Measurements

Neck	Chest	UpperArm	Waist	Hips
in.	in.	in.	in.	in.

Thigh	Calf	Forearm	Weight	Body Fat
in.	in.	in.	in.	%

Resting Heart Rate: - beats per minute -	_____

Date: _____/_____/_____ .... End of 4 Weeks

Notes

Measurements

Neck	Chest	UpperArm	Waist	Hips
in.	in.	in.	in.	in.

Thigh	Calf	Forearm	Weight	Body Fat
in.	in.	in.	in.	%

Resting Heart Rate:
- beats per minute -

Date: _____/_____/_____ _____ End of 8 Week

Notes

Measurements

Neck	Chest	UpperArm	Waist	Hips
in.	in.	in.	in.	in.

Thigh	Calf	Forearm	Weight	Body Fat
in.	in.	in.	in.	%

Resting Heart Rate: - beats per minute -	_____

Date: _____/_____/_____ .... End of 12 Weeks

Notes

_____

_____

_____

_____

_____

_____

_____

_____

_____

_____

_____

_____

_____

_____

_____

_____

Date ___/___/___   Food Log

Meal	Item	Calories	Protein	Fat
Breakfast				
Snack				
Lunch				
Snack				
Dinner				
Snack				
Total				

Notes : _____

_____

_____

_____

_____

_____

_____

_____

_____

DATE:____/____/_____   Muscle's Being Worked

Resistance Training

Exercise	Weight	Sets	Reps	Note

Cardio Training

Type :_____   Time : _____

Type :_____   Time : _____

Notes : _____

_____

_____

_____

Food Log

Meal	Item	Calories	Protein	Fat
Breakfast				
Snack				
Lunch				
Snack				
Dinner				
Snack				
Total				

Notes : _____

_____

_____

_____

_____

_____

_____

_____

_____

_____

ATE:_____/_____/_____   Muscle's Being Worked

Resistance Training

Exercise	Weight	Sets	Reps	Note

Cardio Training

Type :_____ Time : _____

Type :_____ Time : _____

Notes : _____

_____

_____

Date ___/___/____ # Food Log

Meal	Item	Calories	Protein	Fat
Breakfast				
Snack				
Lunch				
Snack				
Dinner				
Snack				
Total				

Notes : _____

_____

_____

_____

_____

_____

_____

_____

_____

DATE:____/____/_____   Muscle's Being Worked

Resistance Training

Exercise	Weight	Sets	Reps	Note

Cardio Training

Type :_____ Time : _____

Type :_____ Time : _____

Notes : _____

_____

_____

Date ___/___/____   # Food Log

Meal	Item	Calories	Protein	Fat
Breakfast				
Snack				
Lunch				
Snack				
Dinner				
Snack				
Total				

Notes : _____

_____
_____
_____
_____
_____
_____
_____
_____
_____

DATE:____/____/_____   Muscle's Being Worked

Resistance Training

Exercise	Weight	Sets	Reps	Note

Cardio Training

Type :_____ Time : _____

Type :_____ Time : _____

Notes : _____

_____

_____

Date ___/___/___   Food Log

Meal	Item	Calories	Protein	Fat
Breakfast				
Snack				
Lunch				
Snack				
Dinner				
Snack				
Total				

Notes : _____

_____

_____

_____

_____

_____

_____

_____

_____

_____

DATE:_____/_____/_____   Muscle's Being Worked

Resistance Training

Exercise	Weight	Sets	Reps	Note

Cardio Training

Type :_____ Time : _____

Type :_____ Time : _____

Notes : _____

_____

_____

Food Log

Meal	Item	Calories	Protein	Fat
Breakfast				
Snack				
Lunch				
Snack				
Dinner				
Snack				
Total				

Notes : _____

_____

_____

_____

_____

_____

_____

_____

_____

_____

DATE:____/____/_____   Muscle's Being Worked

Resistance Training

Exercise	Weight	Sets	Reps	Note

Cardio Training

Type :_____ Time : _____

Type :_____ Time : _____

Notes : _____

_____

_____

Date ___/___/___   Food Log

Meal	Item	Calories	Protein	Fat
Breakfast				
Snack				
Lunch				
Snack				
Dinner				
Snack				
Total				

Notes : _____

_____

_____

_____

_____

_____

_____

_____

_____

_____

DATE:____/____/_____   Muscle's Being Worked

Resistance Training

Exercise	Weight	Sets	Reps	Note

Cardio Training

Type :_____ Time : _____

Type :_____ Time : _____

Notes : _____

_____

_____

Date ___/___/___   Food Log

Meal	Item	Calories	Protein	Fat
Breakfast				
Snack				
Lunch				
Snack				
Dinner				
Snack				
Total				

Notes : _____

_____

_____

_____

_____

_____

_____

_____

_____

_____

ATE:___/___/_____   Muscle's Being Worked

Resistance Training

Exercise	Weight	Sets	Reps	Note

Cardio Training

Type :_____ Time : _____

Type :_____ Time : _____

Notes : _____

_____

_____

_____

Date ___/___/____   # Food Log

Meal	Item	Calories	Protein	Fat
Breakfast				
Snack				
Lunch				
Snack				
Dinner				
Snack				
Total				

Notes : _____

_____

_____

_____

_____

_____

_____

_____

_____

_____

DATE:____/____/_____ Muscle's Being Worked

Resistance Training

Exercise	Weight	Sets	Reps	Note

Cardio Training

Type :_____ Time : _____

Type :_____ Time : _____

Notes : _____

_____

_____

Date ___/___/___   Food Log

Meal	Item	Calories	Protein	Fat
Breakfast				
Snack				
Lunch				
Snack				
Dinner				
Snack				
Total				

Notes : _____

_____

_____

_____

_____

_____

_____

_____

_____

DATE:____/____/_____   Muscle's Being Worked

Resistance Training

Exercise	Weight	Sets	Reps	Note

Cardio Training

Type :_____ Time : _____

Type :_____ Time : _____

Notes : _____

_____

_____

Date ___/___/___   Food Log

Meal	Item	Calories	Protein	Fat
Breakfast				
Snack				
Lunch				
Snack				
Dinner				
Snack				
Total				

Notes : _____

_____

_____

_____

_____

_____

_____

_____

_____

ATE:____/____/_____   Muscle's Being Worked

Resistance Training

Exercise	Weight	Sets	Reps	Note

Cardio Training

Type :_____ Time : _____

Type :_____ Time : _____

Notes : _____

_____

_____

Date ___/___/___   Food Log

Meal	Item	Calories	Protein	Fat
Breakfast				
Snack				
Lunch				
Snack				
Dinner				
Snack				
Total				

Notes : _____

_____

_____

_____

_____

_____

_____

_____

_____

_____

Resistance Training

Exercise	Weight	Sets	Reps	Note

Cardio Training

Type :_____   Time : _____

Type :_____   Time : _____

Notes : _____

_____

_____

Date ___/___/____   Food Log

Meal	Item	Calories	Protein	Fat
Breakfast				
Snack				
Lunch				
Snack				
Dinner				
Snack				
Total				

Notes : _____

_____

_____

_____

_____

_____

_____

_____

_____

DATE:____/____/_____   Muscle's Being Worked

| | | | |

Resistance Training

Exercise	Weight	Sets	Reps	Note

Cardio Training

Type :_____ Time : _____

Type :_____ Time : _____

Notes : _____

_____

_____

Date ___/___/___   Food Log

Meal	Item	Calories	Protein	Fat
Breakfast				
Snack				
Lunch				
Snack				
Dinner				
Snack				
Total				

Notes : _____

_____

_____

_____

_____

_____

_____

_____

_____

DATE:____/____/_____   Muscle's Being Worked

| | | | |

Resistance Training

Exercise	Weight	Sets	Reps	Note

Cardio Training

Type :_____ Time : _____

Type :_____ Time : _____

Notes : _____

_____

_____

Date ___/___/___ Food Log

Meal	Item	Calories	Protein	Fat
Breakfast				
Snack				
Lunch				
Snack				
Dinner				
Snack				
Total				

Notes : _____

_____

_____

_____

_____

_____

_____

_____

_____

DATE:____/____/_____   Muscle's Being Worked

Resistance Training

Exercise	Weight	Sets	Reps	Note

Cardio Training

Type :_____   Time : _____

Type :_____   Time : _____

Notes : _____

_____

_____

Food Log

Meal	Item	Calories	Protein	Fat
Breakfast				
Snack				
Lunch				
Snack				
Dinner				
Snack				
Total				

Notes : _____

_____

_____

_____

_____

_____

_____

_____

_____

DATE:____/____/_____   Muscle's Being Worked

Resistance Training

Exercise	Weight	Sets	Reps	Note

Cardio Training

Type :_____ Time : _____

Type :_____ Time : _____

Notes : _____

_____

_____

Date ___/___/___   Food Log

Meal	Item	Calories	Protein	Fat
Breakfast				
Snack				
Lunch				
Snack				
Dinner				
Snack				
Total				

Notes : _____

_____
_____
_____
_____
_____
_____
_____
_____

ATE:_____/_____/_____   Muscle's Being Worked

Resistance Training

Exercise	Weight	Sets	Reps	Note

Cardio Training

ype :_____ Time : _____

ype :_____ Time : _____

Notes : _____

_____

_____

Date ___/___/___   Food Log

Meal	Item	Calories	Protein	Fat
Breakfast				
Snack				
Lunch				
Snack				
Dinner				
Snack				
Total				

Notes : _____

_____

_____

_____

_____

_____

_____

_____

_____

DATE:____/____/_____   Muscle's Being Worked

| | | | |

Resistance Training

Exercise	Weight	Sets	Reps	Note

Cardio Training

Type :_____ Time : _____

Type :_____ Time : _____

Notes : _____

_____

_____

Date ___/___/___   Food Log

Meal	Item	Calories	Protein	Fat
Breakfast				
Snack				
Lunch				
Snack				
Dinner				
Snack				
Total				

Notes : _____
_____
_____
_____
_____
_____
_____
_____
_____
_____
_____

DATE:_____/_____/_____   Muscle's Being Worked

| | | | |

Resistance Training

Exercise	Weight	Sets	Reps	Note

Cardio Training

Type :_____ Time : _____

Type :_____ Time : _____

Notes : _____

_____

_____

Date ___/___/___   Food Log

Meal	Item	Calories	Protein	Fat
Breakfast				
Snack				
Lunch				
Snack				
Dinner				
Snack				
Total				

Notes : _____

_____

_____

_____

_____

_____

_____

_____

_____

ATE:____/____/_____   Muscle's Being Worked

Resistance Training

Exercise	Weight	Sets	Reps	Note

Cardio Training

Type :_____ Time : _____

Type :_____ Time : _____

Notes : _____

_____

_____

Date ___/___/___   Food Log

Meal	Item	Calories	Protein	Fat
Breakfast				
Snack				
Lunch				
Snack				
Dinner				
Snack				
Total				

Notes : _____

_____

_____

_____

_____

_____

_____

_____

_____

DATE:____/____/_____   Muscle's Being Worked

Resistance Training

Exercise	Weight	Sets	Reps	Note

Cardio Training

Type :_____ Time : _____

Type :_____ Time : _____

Notes : _____

_____

_____

_____

Date ___/___/_____   Food Log

Meal	Item	Calories	Protein	Fat
Breakfast				
Snack				
Lunch				
Snack				
Dinner				
Snack				
Total				

Notes : _____

_____

_____

_____

_____

_____

_____

_____

_____

_____

DATE:____/____/_____   Muscle's Being Worked

Resistance Training

Exercise	Weight	Sets	Reps	Note

Cardio Training

Type :_____ Time : _____

Type :_____ Time : _____

Notes : _____

_____

_____

_____

Date ___/___/____   # Food Log

Meal	Item	Calories	Protein	Fat
Breakfast				
Snack				
Lunch				
Snack				
Dinner				
Snack				
Total				

Notes : _____

_____

_____

_____

_____

_____

_____

_____

_____

ATE:_____/_____/_____   Muscle's Being Worked

Resistance Training

Exercise	Weight	Sets	Reps	Note

Cardio Training

ype :_____ Time : _____

ype :_____ Time : _____

Notes : _____

_____

_____

Food Log

Meal	Item	Calories	Protein	Fat
Breakfast				
Snack				
Lunch				
Snack				
Dinner				
Snack				
Total				

Notes : _____

_____

_____

_____

_____

_____

_____

_____

_____

_____

DATE:____/____/_____   Muscle's Being Worked

Resistance Training

Exercise	Weight	Sets	Reps	Note

Cardio Training

Type :_____ Time : _____

Type :_____ Time : _____

Notes : _____

_____

_____

_____

Food Log

Meal	Item	Calories	Protein	Fat
Breakfast				
Snack				
Lunch				
Snack				
Dinner				
Snack				
Total				

Notes : _____

_____

_____

_____

_____

_____

_____

_____

_____

_____

DATE:_____/_____/_____   Muscle's Being Worked

Resistance Training

Exercise	Weight	Sets	Reps	Note

Cardio Training

Type :_____ Time : _____

Type :_____ Time : _____

Notes : _____

_____

_____

Date ___/___/___   Food Log

Meal	Item	Calories	Protein	Fat
Breakfast				
Snack				
Lunch				
Snack				
Dinner				
Snack				
Total				

Notes : _____

_____

_____

_____

_____

_____

_____

_____

_____

ATE:_____/_____/_____   Muscle's Being Worked

| | | | |

Resistance Training

Exercise	Weight	Sets	Reps	Note

Cardio Training

ype :_____ Time : _____

ype :_____ Time : _____

Notes : _____

_____

_____

Date ___/___/____   Food Log

Meal	Item	Calories	Protein	Fat
Breakfast				
Snack				
Lunch				
Snack				
Dinner				
Snack				
Total				

Notes : _____

_____

_____

_____

_____

_____

_____

_____

_____

Muscle's Being Worked

Resistance Training

Exercise	Weight	Sets	Reps	Note

Cardio Training

Type :_____ Time : _____

Type :_____ Time : _____

Notes : _____

_____

_____

_____

Date ___/___/____   Food Log

Meal	Item	Calories	Protein	Fat
Breakfast				
Snack				
Lunch				
Snack				
Dinner				
Snack				
Total				

Notes : _____

_____

_____

_____

_____

_____

_____

_____

_____

Muscle's Being Worked

Resistance Training

Exercise	Weight	Sets	Reps	Note

Cardio Training

Type :_____ Time : _____

Type :_____ Time : _____

Notes : _____

_____

_____

Date ___/___/____   Food Log

Meal	Item	Calories	Protein	Fat
Breakfast				
Snack				
Lunch				
Snack				
Dinner				
Snack				
Total				

Notes : _____

_____

_____

_____

_____

_____

_____

_____

_____

ATE:____/____/_____   Muscle's Being Worked

| | | | |

Resistance Training

Exercise	Weight	Sets	Reps	Note

Cardio Training

ype :_____ Time : _____

ype :_____ Time : _____

Notes : _____

_____

_____

Date ___/___/___   Food Log

Meal	Item	Calories	Protein	Fat
Breakfast				
Snack				
Lunch				
Snack				
Dinner				
Snack				
Total				

Notes : _____

_____

_____

_____

_____

_____

_____

_____

_____

_____

DATE:_____/_____/_____   Muscle's Being Worked

| | | | |

Resistance Training

Exercise	Weight	Sets	Reps	Note

Cardio Training

Type :_____ Time : _____

Type :_____ Time : _____

Notes : _____

_____

_____

_____

Date ___/___/____   Food Log

Meal	Item	Calories	Protein	Fat
Breakfast				
Snack				
Lunch				
Snack				
Dinner				
Snack				
Total				

Notes : _____

_____

_____

_____

_____

_____

_____

_____

_____

_____

Muscle's Being Worked

Resistance Training

Exercise	Weight	Sets	Reps	Note

Cardio Training

Type :_____   Time : _____

Type :_____   Time : _____

Notes : _____

_____

_____

_____

Date ___/___/___   Food Log

Meal	Item	Calories	Protein	Fat
Breakfast				
Snack				
Lunch				
Snack				
Dinner				
Snack				
Total				

Notes : _____
_____
_____
_____
_____
_____
_____
_____
_____
_____

Resistance Training

Exercise	Weight	Sets	Reps	Note

Cardio Training

ype :_____ Time : _____

ype :_____ Time : _____

Notes : _____

_____

_____

Date ___/___/___   Food Log

Meal	Item	Calories	Protein	Fat
Breakfast				
Snack				
Lunch				
Snack				
Dinner				
Snack				
Total				

Notes : _____

_____

_____

_____

_____

_____

_____

_____

_____

DATE:_____/_____/_____   Muscle's Being Worked

Resistance Training

Exercise	Weight	Sets	Reps	Note

Cardio Training

Type :_____ Time : _____

Type :_____ Time : _____

Notes : _____

_____

_____

Date ___/___/___   Food Log

Meal	Item	Calories	Protein	Fat
Breakfast				
Snack				
Lunch				
Snack				
Dinner				
Snack				
Total				

Notes : _____
_____
_____
_____
_____
_____
_____
_____
_____
_____

DATE:____/____/_____   Muscle's Being Worked

| | | | |

Resistance Training

Exercise	Weight	Sets	Reps	Note
_____	_____	_____	_____	_____
_____	_____	_____	_____	_____
_____	_____	_____	_____	_____
_____	_____	_____	_____	_____
_____	_____	_____	_____	_____
_____	_____	_____	_____	_____
_____	_____	_____	_____	_____
_____	_____	_____	_____	_____
_____	_____	_____	_____	_____
_____	_____	_____	_____	_____
_____	_____	_____	_____	_____
_____	_____	_____	_____	_____
_____	_____	_____	_____	_____
_____	_____	_____	_____	_____
_____	_____	_____	_____	_____
_____	_____	_____	_____	_____
_____	_____	_____	_____	_____
_____	_____	_____	_____	_____
_____	_____	_____	_____	_____

Cardio Training

Type :_____ Time : _____

Type :_____ Time : _____

Notes : _____

_____

_____

Date ___/___/___   # Food Log

Meal	Item	Calories	Protein	Fat
Breakfast				
Snack				
Lunch				
Snack				
Dinner				
Snack				
Total				

Notes : _____

_____

_____

_____

_____

_____

_____

_____

_____

ATE:____/____/_____   Muscle's Being Worked

Resistance Training

Exercise	Weight	Sets	Reps	Note

Cardio Training

ype :_____ Time : _____

ype :_____ Time : _____

Jotes : _____

_____

_____

Date ___/___/____   Food Log

Meal	Item	Calories	Protein	Fat
Breakfast				
Snack				
Lunch				
Snack				
Dinner				
Snack				
Total				

Notes : _____

_____

_____

_____

_____

_____

_____

_____

_____

DATE:____/____/_____   Muscle's Being Worked

| | | | |

Resistance Training

Exercise	Weight	Sets	Reps	Note

Cardio Training

Type :_____ Time : _____

Type :_____ Time : _____

Notes : _____

_____

_____

Food Log

Meal	Item	Calories	Protein	Fat
Breakfast				
Snack				
Lunch				
Snack				
Dinner				
Snack				
Total				

Notes : _____

_____

_____

_____

_____

_____

_____

_____

_____

_____

DATE:____/____/_____ Muscle's Being Worked

Resistance Training

Exercise	Weight	Sets	Reps	Note

Cardio Training

Type :_____ Time : _____

Type :_____ Time : _____

Notes : _____

_____

_____

Date ___/___/___   # Food Log

Meal	Item	Calories	Protein	Fat
Breakfast				
Snack				
Lunch				
Snack				
Dinner				
Snack				
Total				

Notes : _____

_____

_____

_____

_____

_____

_____

_____

_____

ATE:____/____/_____   Muscle's Being Worked

Resistance Training

Exercise	Weight	Sets	Reps	Note

Cardio Training

ype :_____ Time : _____

ype :_____ Time : _____

Notes : _____

_____

_____

Date ___/___/____ Food Log

Meal	Item	Calories	Protein	Fat
Breakfast				
Snack				
Lunch				
Snack				
Dinner				
Snack				
Total				

Notes : _____
_____
_____
_____
_____
_____
_____
_____
_____

DATE:_____/_____/_____   Muscle's Being Worked

Resistance Training

Exercise	Weight	Sets	Reps	Note

Cardio Training

Type :_____   Time : _____

Type :_____   Time : _____

Notes : _____

_____

_____

_____

Date ___/___/___   Food Log

Meal	Item	Calories	Protein	Fat
Breakfast				
Snack				
Lunch				
Snack				
Dinner				
Snack				
Total				

Notes : _____

_____

_____

_____

_____

_____

_____

_____

_____

_____

DATE:____/____/_____   Muscle's Being Worked

Resistance Training

Exercise	Weight	Sets	Reps	Note

Cardio Training

Type :_____   Time : _____

Type :_____   Time : _____

Notes : _____

_____

_____

_____

Date ___/___/___   # Food Log

Meal	Item	Calories	Protein	Fat
Breakfast				
Snack				
Lunch				
Snack				
Dinner				
Snack				
Total				

Notes : _____

_____
_____
_____
_____
_____
_____
_____
_____

ATE:____/____/_____   Muscle's Being Worked

| | | | |

Resistance Training

Exercise	Weight	Sets	Reps	Note

Cardio Training

ype :_____ Time : _____

ype :_____ Time : _____

Iotes : _____

_____

_____

Food Log

Meal	Item	Calories	Protein	Fat
Breakfast				
Snack				
Lunch				
Snack				
Dinner				
Snack				
Total				

Notes : _____

_____

_____

_____

_____

_____

_____

_____

_____

DATE:_____/_____/_____ Muscle's Being Worked

Resistance Training

Exercise	Weight	Sets	Reps	Note

Cardio Training

Type :_____ Time : _____

Type :_____ Time : _____

Notes : _____

_____

_____

Food Log

Meal	Item	Calories	Protein	Fat
Breakfast				
Snack				
Lunch				
Snack				
Dinner				
Snack				
Total				

Notes : _____

_____

_____

_____

_____

_____

_____

_____

_____

_____

DATE:____/____/_____   Muscle's Being Worked

Resistance Training

Exercise	Weight	Sets	Reps	Note

Cardio Training

Type :_____ Time : _____

Type :_____ Time : _____

Notes : _____

_____

_____

_____

Date ___/___/___   Food Log

Meal	Item	Calories	Protein	Fat
Breakfast				
Snack				
Lunch				
Snack				
Dinner				
Snack				
Total				

Notes : _____

_____

_____

_____

_____

_____

_____

_____

_____

Resistance Training

Exercise	Weight	Sets	Reps	Note

Cardio Training

ype :_____ Time : _____

ype :_____ Time : _____

Jotes : _____

_____

_____

_____

Date ___/___/___   Food Log

Meal	Item	Calories	Protein	Fat
Breakfast				
Snack				
Lunch				
Snack				
Dinner				
Snack				
Total				

Notes : _____

_____

_____

_____

_____

_____

_____

_____

_____

DATE:_____/_____/_____   Muscle's Being Worked

Resistance Training

Exercise	Weight	Sets	Reps	Note

Cardio Training

Type :_____ Time : _____

Type :_____ Time : _____

Notes : _____

_____

_____

Food Log

Meal	Item	Calories	Protein	Fat
Breakfast				
Snack				
Lunch				
Snack				
Dinner				
Snack				
Total				

Notes : _____

_____

_____

_____

_____

_____

_____

_____

_____

DATE:____/____/_____   Muscle's Being Worked

| | | | |

Resistance Training

Exercise	Weight	Sets	Reps	Note

Cardio Training

Type :_____ Time : _____

Type :_____ Time : _____

Notes : _____

_____

_____

Date ___/___/____   Food Log

Meal	Item	Calories	Protein	Fat
Breakfast				
Snack				
Lunch				
Snack				
Dinner				
Snack				
Total				

Notes : _____

_____

_____

_____

_____

_____

_____

_____

_____

_____

ATE:_____/_____/_____   Muscle's Being Worked

Resistance Training

Exercise	Weight	Sets	Reps	Note

Cardio Training

ype :_____ Time : _____

ype :_____ Time : _____

Iotes : _____

_____

_____

Food Log

Meal	Item	Calories	Protein	Fat
Breakfast				
Snack				
Lunch				
Snack				
Dinner				
Snack				
Total				

Notes : _____

_____

_____

_____

_____

_____

_____

_____

_____

DATE:____/____/_____   Muscle's Being Worked

Resistance Training

Exercise	Weight	Sets	Reps	Note

Cardio Training

Type :_____ Time : _____

Type :_____ Time : _____

Notes : _____

_____

_____

Date ___/___/___   Food Log

Meal	Item	Calories	Protein	Fat
Breakfast				
Snack				
Lunch				
Snack				
Dinner				
Snack				
Total				

Notes : _____
_____
_____
_____
_____
_____
_____
_____
_____
_____

DATE:_____/_____/_____ Muscle's Being Worked

Resistance Training

Exercise	Weight	Sets	Reps	Note

Cardio Training

Type :_____ Time : _____

Type :_____ Time : _____

Notes : _____

_____

_____

Date ___/___/___   Food Log

Meal	Item	Calories	Protein	Fat
Breakfast				
Snack				
Lunch				
Snack				
Dinner				
Snack				
Total				

Notes : _____

_____

_____

_____

_____

_____

_____

_____

_____

ATE:____/____/_____   Muscle's Being Worked

Resistance Training

Exercise	Weight	Sets	Reps	Note

Cardio Training

ype :_____ Time : _____

ype :_____ Time : _____

Jotes : _____

_____

_____

Food Log

Meal	Item	Calories	Protein	Fat
Breakfast				
Snack				
Lunch				
Snack				
Dinner				
Snack				
Total				

Notes : _____

_____

_____

_____

_____

_____

_____

_____

_____

DATE:____/____/_____   Muscle's Being Worked

Resistance Training

Exercise	Weight	Sets	Reps	Note

Cardio Training

Type :_____ Time : _____

Type :_____ Time : _____

Notes : _____

_____

_____

Date ___/___/___   Food Log

Meal	Item	Calories	Protein	Fat
Breakfast				
Snack				
Lunch				
Snack				
Dinner				
Snack				
Total				

Notes : _____

_____

_____

_____

_____

_____

_____

_____

_____

_____

Muscle's Being Worked

Resistance Training

Exercise	Weight	Sets	Reps	Note

Cardio Training

Type :_____ Time : _____

Type :_____ Time : _____

Notes : _____

_____

_____

Date ___/___/___   Food Log

Meal	Item	Calories	Protein	Fat
Breakfast				
Snack				
Lunch				
Snack				
Dinner				
Snack				
Total				

Notes : _____

_____

_____

_____

_____

_____

_____

_____

_____

_____

ATE:____/____/_____   Muscle's Being Worked

Resistance Training

Exercise	Weight	Sets	Reps	Note

Cardio Training

ype :_____ Time : _____

ype :_____ Time : _____

Iotes : _____

_____

_____

Date ___/___/___   Food Log

Meal	Item	Calories	Protein	Fat
Breakfast				
Snack				
Lunch				
Snack				
Dinner				
Snack				
Total				

Notes : _____

_____

_____

_____

_____

_____

_____

_____

_____

_____

DATE:____/____/_____   Muscle's Being Worked

| | | | |

Resistance Training

Exercise	Weight	Sets	Reps	Note

Cardio Training

Type :_____ Time : _____

Type :_____ Time : _____

Notes : _____

_____

_____

Date ___/___/___   Food Log

Meal	Item	Calories	Protein	Fat
Breakfast				
Snack				
Lunch				
Snack				
Dinner				
Snack				
Total				

Notes : _____

_____

_____

_____

_____

_____

_____

_____

_____

DATE:_____/_____/_____   Muscle's Being Worked

Resistance Training

Exercise	Weight	Sets	Reps	Note

Cardio Training

Type :_____ Time : _____

Type :_____ Time : _____

Notes : _____

_____

_____

Date ___/___/___   Food Log

Meal	Item	Calories	Protein	Fat
Breakfast				
Snack				
Lunch				
Snack				
Dinner				
Snack				
Total				

Notes : _____

_____
_____
_____
_____
_____
_____
_____
_____

ATE:_____/_____/_____   Muscle's Being Worked

Resistance Training

Exercise	Weight	Sets	Reps	Note

Cardio Training

ype :_____   Time : _____

ype :_____   Time : _____

Jotes : _____

_____

_____

Date ___/___/___   Food Log

Meal	Item	Calories	Protein	Fat
Breakfast				
Snack				
Lunch				
Snack				
Dinner				
Snack				
Total				

Notes : _____

_____

_____

_____

_____

_____

_____

_____

_____

DATE:_____/_____/_____   Muscle's Being Worked

| | | | |

Resistance Training

Exercise	Weight	Sets	Reps	Note

Cardio Training

Type :_____ Time : _____

Type :_____ Time : _____

Notes : _____

_____

_____

Date ___/___/___   Food Log

Meal	Item	Calories	Protein	Fat
Breakfast				
Snack				
Lunch				
Snack				
Dinner				
Snack				
Total				

Notes : _____
_____
_____
_____
_____
_____
_____
_____
_____

DATE:____/____/_____   Muscle's Being Worked

| | | | |

Resistance Training

Exercise	Weight	Sets	Reps	Note

Cardio Training

Type :_____ Time : _____

Type :_____ Time : _____

Notes : _____

_____

_____

Date ___/___/___   Food Log

Meal	Item	Calories	Protein	Fat
Breakfast				
Snack				
Lunch				
Snack				
Dinner				
Snack				
Total				

Notes : _____

_____

_____

_____

_____

_____

_____

_____

_____

ATE:____/____/_____   Muscle's Being Worked

| | | | |

Resistance Training

Exercise	Weight	Sets	Reps	Note

Cardio Training

ype :_____ Time : _____

ype :_____ Time : _____

Jotes : _____

_____

_____

Food Log

Date ___/___/___

Meal	Item	Calories	Protein	Fat
Breakfast				
Snack				
Lunch				
Snack				
Dinner				
Snack				
Total				

Notes : _____

_____

_____

_____

_____

_____

_____

_____

DATE:____/____/_____   Muscle's Being Worked

Resistance Training

Exercise	Weight	Sets	Reps	Note

Cardio Training

Type :_____ Time : _____

Type :_____ Time : _____

Notes : _____

_____

_____

Date ___/___/___   Food Log

Meal	Item	Calories	Protein	Fat
Breakfast				
Snack				
Lunch				
Snack				
Dinner				
Snack				
Total				

Notes : _____
_____
_____
_____
_____
_____
_____
_____
_____
_____

DATE:____/____/_____ Muscle's Being Worked

Resistance Training

Exercise	Weight	Sets	Reps	Note

Cardio Training

Type :_____ Time : _____

Type :_____ Time : _____

Notes : _____

Date ___/___/___   Food Log

Meal	Item	Calories	Protein	Fat
Breakfast				
Snack				
Lunch				
Snack				
Dinner				
Snack				
Total				

Notes : _____

_____

_____

_____

_____

_____

_____

_____

_____

ATE:____/____/_____   Muscle's Being Worked

Resistance Training

Exercise	Weight	Sets	Reps	Note

Cardio Training

ype :_____ Time : _____

ype :_____ Time : _____

Jotes : _____

_____

_____

Food Log

Meal	Item	Calories	Protein	Fat
Breakfast				
Snack				
Lunch				
Snack				
Dinner				
Snack				
Total				

Notes : _____

_____

_____

_____

_____

_____

_____

_____

DATE:_____/_____/_____   Muscle's Being Worked

Resistance Training

Exercise	Weight	Sets	Reps	Note

Cardio Training

Type :_____ Time : _____

Type :_____ Time : _____

Notes : _____

_____

_____

Date ___/___/____   Food Log

Meal	Item	Calories	Protein	Fat
Breakfast				
Snack				
Lunch				
Snack				
Dinner				
Snack				
Total				

Notes : _____

_____

_____

_____

_____

_____

_____

_____

_____

DATE:____/____/_____   Muscle's Being Worked

| | | | |

Resistance Training

Exercise	Weight	Sets	Reps	Note

Cardio Training

Type :_____ Time : _____

Type :_____ Time : _____

Notes : _____

_____

_____

Date ___/___/____   # Food Log

Meal	Item	Calories	Protein	Fat
Breakfast				
Snack				
Lunch				
Snack				
Dinner				
Snack				
Total				

Notes : _____

_____

_____

_____

_____

_____

_____

_____

_____

ATE:____/____/_____   Muscle's Being Worked

| | | | |

Resistance Training

Exercise	Weight	Sets	Reps	Note

Cardio Training

ype :_____ Time : _____

ype :_____ Time : _____

Iotes : _____

_____

_____

Food Log

Meal	Item	Calories	Protein	Fat
Breakfast				
Snack				
Lunch				
Snack				
Dinner				
Snack				
Total				

Notes : _____

_____

_____

_____

_____

_____

_____

_____

_____

DATE:____/____/_____   Muscle's Being Worked

Resistance Training

Exercise	Weight	Sets	Reps	Note

Cardio Training

Type :_____ Time : _____

Type :_____ Time : _____

Notes : _____

_____

_____

Meal	Item	Calories	Protein	Fat
Breakfast				
Snack				
Lunch				
Snack				
Dinner				
Snack				
Total				

Notes : _____

_____

_____

_____

_____

_____

_____

_____

_____

_____

DATE:____/____/_____   Muscle's Being Worked

Resistance Training

Exercise	Weight	Sets	Reps	Note

Cardio Training

Type :_____ Time : _____

Type :_____ Time : _____

Notes : _____

_____

_____

Date ___/___/___   Food Log

Meal	Item	Calories	Protein	Fat
Breakfast				
Snack				
Lunch				
Snack				
Dinner				
Snack				
Total				

Notes : _____

_____

_____

_____

_____

_____

_____

_____

_____

ATE:____/____/_____   Muscle's Being Worked

| | | | |

Resistance Training

Exercise	Weight	Sets	Reps	Note

Cardio Training

ype :_____ Time : _____

ype :_____ Time : _____

Iotes : _____

_____

_____

Date ___/___/____   Food Log

Meal	Item	Calories	Protein	Fat
Breakfast				
Snack				
Lunch				
Snack				
Dinner				
Snack				
Total				

Notes : _____

_____
_____
_____
_____
_____
_____
_____
_____
_____

DATE:____/____/_____   Muscle's Being Worked

| | | | |

Resistance Training

Exercise	Weight	Sets	Reps	Note

Cardio Training

Type :_____   Time : _____

Type :_____   Time : _____

Notes : _____

_____

_____

_____

Date ___/___/____   # Food Log

Meal	Item	Calories	Protein	Fat
Breakfast				
Snack				
Lunch				
Snack				
Dinner				
Snack				
Total				

Notes : _____

_____

_____

_____

_____

_____

_____

_____

_____

_____

DATE:_____/_____/_____   Muscle's Being Worked

| | | | |

Resistance Training

Exercise	Weight	Sets	Reps	Note

Cardio Training

Type :_____ Time : _____

Type :_____ Time : _____

Notes : _____

_____

_____

Date ___/___/___   Food Log

Meal	Item	Calories	Protein	Fat
Breakfast				
Snack				
Lunch				
Snack				
Dinner				
Snack				
Total				

Notes : _____

_____

_____

_____

_____

_____

_____

_____

_____

ATE:____/____/_____   Muscle's Being Worked

| | | | |

Resistance Training

Exercise	Weight	Sets	Reps	Note

Cardio Training

ype :_____ Time : _____

ype :_____ Time : _____

Jotes : _____

_____

_____

Date ___/___/___   # Food Log

Meal	Item	Calories	Protein	Fat
Breakfast				
Snack				
Lunch				
Snack				
Dinner				
Snack				
Total				

Notes : _____

_____
_____
_____
_____
_____
_____
_____
_____

DATE:____/____/_____ Muscle's Being Worked

Resistance Training

Exercise	Weight	Sets	Reps	Note

Cardio Training

Type :_____ Time : _____

Type :_____ Time : _____

Notes : _____

_____

_____

Date ___/___/____   Food Log

Meal	Item	Calories	Protein	Fat
Breakfast				
Snack				
Lunch				
Snack				
Dinner				
Snack				
Total				

Notes : _____

_____

_____

_____

_____

_____

_____

_____

_____

_____

DATE:____/____/_____   Muscle's Being Worked

Resistance Training

Exercise	Weight	Sets	Reps	Note

Cardio Training

Type :_____   Time : _____

Type :_____   Time : _____

Notes : _____

_____

_____

Date ___/___/___   Food Log

Meal	Item	Calories	Protein	Fat
Breakfast				
Snack				
Lunch				
Snack				
Dinner				
Snack				
Total				

Notes : _____

_____

_____

_____

_____

_____

_____

_____

_____

ATE:_____/_____/_____   Muscle's Being Worked

Resistance Training

Exercise	Weight	Sets	Reps	Note

Cardio Training

ype :_____ Time : _____

ype :_____ Time : _____

Notes : _____

_____

_____

_____

Date ___/___/___   Food Log

Meal	Item	Calories	Protein	Fat
Breakfast				
Snack				
Lunch				
Snack				
Dinner				
Snack				
Total				

Notes : _____

_____

_____

_____

_____

_____

_____

_____

_____

_____

DATE:____/____/_____   Muscle's Being Worked

Resistance Training

Exercise	Weight	Sets	Reps	Note

Cardio Training

Type :_____ Time : _____

Type :_____ Time : _____

Notes : _____

_____

_____

Food Log

Meal	Item	Calories	Protein	Fat
Breakfast				
Snack				
Lunch				
Snack				
Dinner				
Snack				
Total				

Notes : _____

_____

_____

_____

_____

_____

_____

_____

_____

_____

DATE:____/____/_____   Muscle's Being Worked

Resistance Training

Exercise	Weight	Sets	Reps	Note

Cardio Training

Type :_____ Time : _____

Type :_____ Time : _____

Notes : _____

_____

_____

Date ___/___/___   # Food Log

Meal	Item	Calories	Protein	Fat
Breakfast				
Snack				
Lunch				
Snack				
Dinner				
Snack				
Total				

Notes : _____

_____

_____

_____

_____

_____

_____

_____

_____

_____

ATE:_____/_____/_____   Muscle's Being Worked

| | | | |

Resistance Training

Exercise	Weight	Sets	Reps	Note

Cardio Training

ype :_____ Time : _____

ype :_____ Time : _____

Notes : _____

_____

_____

Food Log

Meal	Item	Calories	Protein	Fat
Breakfast				
Snack				
Lunch				
Snack				
Dinner				
Snack				
Total				

Notes : _____

_____

_____

_____

_____

_____

_____

_____

_____

DATE:____/____/_____   Muscle's Being Worked

Resistance Training

Exercise	Weight	Sets	Reps	Note

Cardio Training

Type :_____ Time : _____

Type :_____ Time : _____

Notes : _____

_____

_____

Date ___/___/____   Food Log

Meal	Item	Calories	Protein	Fat
Breakfast				
Snack				
Lunch				
Snack				
Dinner				
Snack				
Total				

Notes : _____

_____

_____

_____

_____

_____

_____

_____

_____

DATE:____/____/_____   Muscle's Being Worked

Resistance Training

Exercise	Weight	Sets	Reps	Note

Cardio Training

Type :_____ Time : _____

Type :_____ Time : _____

Notes : _____

_____

_____

Date ___/___/___   Food Log

Meal	Item	Calories	Protein	Fat
Breakfast				
Snack				
Lunch				
Snack				
Dinner				
Snack				
Total				

Notes : _____

_____
_____
_____
_____
_____
_____
_____
_____
_____

DATE:_____/_____/_____   Muscle's Being Worked

Resistance Training

Exercise	Weight	Sets	Reps	Note

Cardio Training

Type :_____ Time : _____

Type :_____ Time : _____

Notes : _____

_____

_____

_____

Date ___/___/___ Food Log

Meal	Item	Calories	Protein	Fat
Breakfast				
Snack				
Lunch				
Snack				
Dinner				
Snack				
Total				

Notes : _____

_____

_____

_____

_____

_____

_____

_____

_____

DATE:____/____/_____   Muscle's Being Worked

Resistance Training

Exercise	Weight	Sets	Reps	Note

Cardio Training

Type :_____ Time : _____

Type :_____ Time : _____

Notes : _____

_____

_____

_____

Food Log

Meal	Item	Calories	Protein	Fat
Breakfast				
Snack				
Lunch				
Snack				
Dinner				
Snack				
Total				

Notes : _____

_____

_____

_____

_____

_____

_____

_____

_____

_____

DATE:_____/_____/_____   Muscle's Being Worked

Resistance Training

Exercise	Weight	Sets	Reps	Note

Cardio Training

Type :_____ Time : _____

Type :_____ Time : _____

Notes : _____

_____

_____

Date ___/___/___   # Food Log

Meal	Item	Calories	Protein	Fat
Breakfast				
Snack				
Lunch				
Snack				
Dinner				
Snack				
Total				

Notes : _____
_____
_____
_____
_____
_____
_____
_____
_____

ATE:____/____/_____   Muscle's Being Worked

| | | | |

Resistance Training

Exercise	Weight	Sets	Reps	Note

Cardio Training

ype :_____ Time : _____

ype :_____ Time : _____

lotes : _____

_____

_____

Date ___/___/___   Food Log

Meal	Item	Calories	Protein	Fat
Breakfast				
Snack				
Lunch				
Snack				
Dinner				
Snack				
Total				

Notes : _____

_____

_____

_____

_____

_____

_____

_____

_____

DATE:____/____/_____   Muscle's Being Worked

Resistance Training

Exercise	Weight	Sets	Reps	Note

Cardio Training

Type :_____ Time : _____

Type :_____ Time : _____

Notes : _____

_____

_____

Food Log

Meal	Item	Calories	Protein	Fat
Breakfast				
Snack				
Lunch				
Snack				
Dinner				
Snack				
Total				

Notes : _____

_____

_____

_____

_____

_____

_____

_____

_____

_____

Resistance Training

Exercise	Weight	Sets	Reps	Note

Cardio Training

Type :_____   Time : _____

Type :_____   Time : _____

Notes : _____

_____

_____

Date ___/___/___   Food Log

Meal	Item	Calories	Protein	Fat
Breakfast				
Snack				
Lunch				
Snack				
Dinner				
Snack				
Total				

Notes : _____

_____

_____

_____

_____

_____

_____

_____

_____

_____

ATE:____/____/_____   Muscle's Being Worked

Resistance Training

Exercise	Weight	Sets	Reps	Note

Cardio Training

ype :_____ Time : _____

ype :_____ Time : _____

Jotes : _____

_____

_____

Date ___/___/___   # Food Log

Meal	Item	Calories	Protein	Fat
Breakfast				
Snack				
Lunch				
Snack				
Dinner				
Snack				
Total				

Notes : _____

_____

_____

_____

_____

_____

_____

_____

_____

DATE:____/____/_____   Muscle's Being Worked

Resistance Training

Exercise	Weight	Sets	Reps	Note

Cardio Training

Type :_____ Time : _____

Type :_____ Time : _____

Notes : _____

_____

_____

Date ___/___/___   Food Log

Meal	Item	Calories	Protein	Fat
Breakfast				
Snack				
Lunch				
Snack				
Dinner				
Snack				
Total				

Notes : _____

_____

_____

_____

_____

_____

_____

_____

_____

_____

DATE:_____/_____/_____   Muscle's Being Worked

| | | | |

Resistance Training

Exercise	Weight	Sets	Reps	Note

Cardio Training

Type :_____ Time : _____

Type :_____ Time : _____

Notes : _____

_____

_____

Date ___/___/___ Food Log

Meal	Item	Calories	Protein	Fat
Breakfast				
Snack				
Lunch				
Snack				
Dinner				
Snack				
Total				

Notes : _____

_____

_____

_____

_____

_____

_____

_____

_____

_____

DATE:_____/_____/_____   Muscle's Being Worked

Resistance Training

Exercise	Weight	Sets	Reps	Note

Cardio Training

Type :_____ Time : _____

Type :_____ Time : _____

Notes : _____

_____

_____

This Training Log Belongs To:

_____

If Found Please Return To:

_____
_____
_____
_____
_____

If you would like a personalized diet
or exercise program
send me an email
wilberto.burgos@yahoo.com

www.ingramcontent.com/pod-product-compliance
Lightning Source LLC
Chambersburg PA
CBHW061407280526
45784CB00001B/400